Somatic Therapy
For Beginners
Self-Soothing Techniques, A DIY Guide to
Healing Trauma, Enhancing the Mind-Body
Connection, and Relieving Stress with
Somatic Psychotherapy.

Title:
Somatic Therapy
For Beginners

Subtitle
Self-Soothing Techniques, A DIY Guide to
Healing Trauma, Enhancing the Mind-Body
Connection, and Relieving Stress with
Somatic Psychotherapy.

Copyright © 2023 by (Cora Ebert)

Printed in the United States of America.

ISBN: 9798869960146

TABLE OF CONTENT

INTRODUCTION

The search for comprehensive well-being has motivated many people to investigate alternate methods of treatment in this fast-paced and sometimes chaotic environment that we inhabit. Somatic therapy has emerged as a deep and transforming method. It provides a one-of-a-kind lens through which individuals may connect with their inner selves, which in turn fosters healing from the inside out. The purpose of this introduction is to offer a thorough summary of somatic therapy by digging into its core ideas and the complex dynamic that exists between the body and the mind.

Understanding Somatic Therapy

Somatic Therapy is a method that, at its most fundamental level, acknowledges the natural link that exists between the human body and the human mind. Somatic therapy, in contrast to more conventional therapeutic approaches, which may concentrate largely on verbal communication, values the knowledge that is held inside the body. It recognizes that events, particularly traumatic ones, are not just etched in one's mind but are also stored in the tissues, muscles, and neurological system of one's body as well as being imprinted in one's memory.

The idea upon which somatic therapy is based is that the human body is a repository of knowledge and a live record of our experiences throughout life. The goal of practitioners of somatic therapy is to excavate and process unresolved feelings, memories, and traumas that may be deeply ingrained in the body via the use of gentle exploration and heightened awareness of the sensations that occur in the body. This knowledge of the body as a reservoir of lived experiences lays the groundwork for a therapeutic journey that extends beyond the boundaries of conventional talk therapy.

Overview of the Body-Mind Connection

The idea that there is a connection between the body and the mind is fundamental to the practice of somatic therapy. This connection emphasizes the complicated and two-way interaction that exists between one's bodily experiences and their emotional well-being. This relationship questions the traditional dichotomy between the mind and the body by presenting them as complementary but interdependent aspects of a single whole. It is a fundamental tenet of somatic therapy to acknowledge that any shift in a client's physical or emotional state will invariably affect other facets of their being.

The concept that there is a link between the body and the mind is not a new one; in fact, ancient healing practices from a variety of cultures have recognized this interdependence for a very long time. Somatic therapy, on the other hand, offers a modern and scientifically informed framework that may be utilized to investigate and make use of this link for therapeutic objectives.

Take, for instance, the feeling of being under pressure or stress. In conventional settings, the mental or emotional condition is typically considered to be the defining characteristic of stress. On the other hand, the theory of somatic therapy proposes that stress may have an effect not just on the mind but also on the body. Tension in the muscles changed breathing patterns, and other bodily signs are all possible outcomes of prolonged exposure to stress. On the other hand, one may favorably affect the emotional and mental components of well-being by treating these bodily manifestations through somatic therapies.

Foundations of Somatic Therapy

It is necessary to investigate the roots of somatic therapy to fully appreciate its breadth and complexity. Somatic Therapy is a multidisciplinary approach that integrates concepts from body-oriented therapies, psychology, and neuroscience. Peter A. Levine is considered one of the pioneers of somatic therapy, having developed somatic Experiencing via his ground-breaking research in the 1970s.

A fundamental component of somatic therapy, somatic Experiencing focuses on using the body's inherent knowledge to reframe and heal trauma. Techniques for

Somatic Experiencing were developed in response to Levine's studies of the animal realm, namely how animals naturally release surplus energy following a life-threatening experience.

Wilhelm Reich, a psychotherapist who studied the relationship between physical and emotional health, is another significant figure. Reich's theory of "body armor" emphasizes how emotional strain and trauma may lodge physically in the body, resulting in long-term patterns of restriction and tension. Reich's ideas are incorporated into and expanded upon by somatic therapy, which provides useful techniques for releasing and processing these pent-up tensions.

Together with these core concepts, body-centered psychotherapy, mindfulness exercises, and other somatic disciplines like dance and yoga are all incorporated into somatic therapy. The discipline is enhanced by this multidisciplinary approach, which offers a wide range of instruments to meet the specific requirements and desires of those looking to recover via somatic exploration.

Fundamentally, Somatic Therapy is predicated on the idea that the body is an active partner in the healing process rather than only a passive conduit for the mind. People can get deep insights and initiate life-changing change by becoming aware of and receptive to their bodies cues.

In the parts that follow, we will examine the fundamental ideas of somatic therapy in more detail, revealing how practitioners work with the body-mind link to promote healing and well-being. Through the use of basic methods to more complex applications, Somatic Therapy offers a route to self-realization, fortitude, and a closer relationship with the body's innate knowledge.

HISTORICAL ROOTS AND DEVELOPMENT

The origins of somatic therapy may be traced back far into the history of both psychological and somatic research. This treatment places a significant focus on the delicate dance that takes place between the body and the mind. This trip through history sheds light on the development of somatic practices, the maturation of theoretical frameworks, and the fundamental principles that serve as the basis for body-centered approaches to healing.

Theoretical Frameworks

• *Early Explorations and Influences*

The historical beginnings of somatic therapy may be traced back to the pioneers who paved the way for a better understanding of the dynamic relationship that exists between the mind and the body. Wilhelm Reich, a psychoanalyst who worked in the early to middle of the 20th century, was a significant contributor to the formation of early somatic notions. Reich was the first to propose the concept of "body armor," which postulates that the human body stores tension as well as memories of emotional events, which can result in physical symptoms of psychological discomfort.

The work done by Reich motivated succeeding generations of therapists to investigate how the body and mind may be integrated into therapeutic procedures. The second half of the 20th century, on the other hand, was the period during which Somatic Therapy first started to develop into its unique field.

- **Development of Somatic Experiencing**

The birth of somatic experiencing is widely regarded as one of the most significant turning points in the history of somatic therapy (SE). Dr. Peter A. Levine, a clinical psychologist and biologist, established SE in the 1970s. He was inspired to create the

13

practice by his studies of the animal kingdom and their innate capacity to deal with and recover from traumatic experiences. Because Levine understood the value of treating trauma not just via verbal discourse but also through the body's intrinsic power to heal, his work represents a paradigm change in therapeutic techniques. This shift was brought about as a result of Levine's work.

Core Principles of Somatic Experiencing

- *Somatic Experiencing as a Trauma Resolution Model*

Somatic therapy is based on the basic concept of somatic experiencing, which acts as a guide for comprehending traumatic experiences and finding effective ways to overcome their effects. According to the SE model, trauma is seen to be imperfect bodily reactions to situations that are both overwhelming and life-threatening. These inadequate reactions, which are frequently preserved in the body, can be the root cause of a wide variety of physical and mental disorders.

Facilitating the completion of these incomplete bodily reactions is at the heart of the key ideas that underpin Somatic Experiencing (SE). The idea of titration, in which the therapist leads the patient through slow and controlled explorations of the bodily feelings linked with traumatic experiences, is fundamental to this method. The body is given the space and support it needs to release pent-up energy when the process of titrating is carried out. This results in a better-regulated neurological system and a sense of resolve.

- *Somatic Experiencing Techniques*

In the process of healing, Somatic Experiencing makes use of several different approaches to tap into the body's intrinsic wisdom. Activities that focus on building a sense of safety and connection with the present moment are frequently used to begin sessions. These exercises are typically called grounding exercises. The clients are helped to become more conscious of the sensations that are occurring throughout their bodies, which encourages a careful investigation of the felt sense.

Pendulation is an important part of Somatic Experiencing; it is a process that entails going between the activation of traumatic memories and the sense of safety and resourcefulness. Pendulation is an important component of Somatic Experiencing. The individual can progressively discharge and gain control over the overpowering emotions linked with the trauma via the use of this rhythmic exercise.

Following the client's physiological and sensory reactions to recognize and treat small alterations in the nervous system is the task of tracking, which is a skill that may be improved via the practice of somatic experiencing (SE). A client's connection with traumatic memories and sensations can be renegotiated with the help of a therapist if they track the client's responses to these sensations and recollections.

Somatic Experiencing is an approach that utilizes these and other methods to help people who have been through traumatic experiences regain a sense of safety, resilience, and empowerment within themselves. Somatic Experiencing stands out from more standard talk treatments in that it incorporates body-centered techniques. This makes it an innovative and very successful means of achieving therapeutic goals.

The Body as a Gateway to Healing

- ***Embodied Wisdom and Unconscious Processes***

The idea that one's physical self may act as a portal to one's emotional and spiritual well-being is fundamental to the origins and evolution of the field of somatic therapy. The traditional approach to psychoanalysis frequently concentrates on investigating the conscious mind, while putting the body and the processes occurring inside it in the background. Somatic therapy, on the other hand, acknowledges that the body is a storehouse of knowledge and that it is the keeper of the key that will open unconscious content.

People place a high value on the information that may be gleaned from the reactions, sensations, and expressions of the body. Subtle alterations in breathing patterns, for instance, might point to the presence of underlying emotional states. Chronic patterns of tension, on the other hand, may point to areas of unresolved trauma. Individuals and therapists both can access deeper levels of experience, which may not be easily available through verbal communication alone if they attune themselves to the signals their bodies are sending them.

- *Integration of Mindfulness and Body Awareness*

The practices of mindfulness and body awareness are given a significant amount of weight in somatic therapy as therapeutic tools. Individuals are encouraged to build an awareness of their experience in the present moment that is free from judgment via the practice of mindfulness, which has its origins in ancient contemplative traditions. When applied to the body, mindfulness transforms into a potent instrument that enables one to observe sensations, emotions, and thinking patterns without becoming attached to or avoiding them.

Individuals learn to be present with their bodily sensations via the practice of body awareness, which enables them to conduct a more in-depth investigation of the terrain that lies within themselves. This heightened awareness helps people connect with the now and now, which grounds them in their body experience and makes it easier for them to let go of built-up tension and stress.

- **The Role of Movement and Expression**

Movement and expression as means of self-healing are fundamental components of somatic therapy, which recognizes both as essential to the therapeutic process. Utilizing the body's inherent drive for motion as a method for releasing pent-up energy, alleviating muscle tension, and fostering a feeling of vigor is the goal of many forms of exercise. Movement, whether it be via

23

moderate exercises, dancing, or the expressive arts, becomes a language through which the body interacts with the outside world and processes the experiences it has had.

Individuals have the option to verbalize their feelings and sensations when they express themselves through expressive modalities. This kind of non-verbal communication makes it possible for the knowledge of the body to be expressed in a manner that is both direct and unfiltered. When people express themselves via movement and creativity, they may find themselves opening up to new facets of their experience, which can ultimately result in a closer connection that is more integrated and harmonious with their body.

BODY AWARENESS AND MINDFULNESS

When it comes to the practice of somatic therapy, the twin pillars of body awareness and mindfulness serve as guiding lights, illuminating the way toward healing and self-discovery. This investigation dives into the complicated terrain of body memory, the subtle world of sensations and emotions, and the essential strategies used in Somatic Therapy to establish a profound connection with the body-mind complex in order to achieve the purpose of the therapy.

- ***Unpacking Body Memory***

The Living Archive Within

Recognizing the body as a living archive of our experiences is a fundamental component of somatic therapy, which makes unpacking body memory a vital part of the practice. In contrast to explicit memories, which are stored in the brain and may be retrieved at any time, body memories are stored in the tissues, muscles, and nervous system and are not always accessible to conscious consciousness. These recollections might have been sparked by a wide variety of situations, ranging from happy occasions to distressing occurrences.

Unresolved experiences, particularly traumatic ones, can get entrenched in the body, impacting patterns of movement, posture, and even the way we breathe. This is one of the tenets of somatic therapy, which recognizes this phenomenon. The process of unpacking body memory entails bringing these implicit memories into conscious consciousness, which enables people to investigate and let go of the physical impressions left by previous events.

Embodied Trauma and Healing

In the framework of somatics, trauma is not something that is restricted to the mind but rather something that permeates the fundamental fabric of the body. Take, for example, a person who has been in a vehicle accident; their body may retain the memory of the hit, which can lead to ongoing tension, discomfort, or changed movement patterns. To unpack this bodily memory, individuals need to be carefully guided to become attuned to the sensations that are connected with the traumatic experience.

The practice of Somatic Therapy, in particular the approaches that have evolved from Somatic Experiencing, emphasizes taking a titrated approach to investigating bodily memory. Titrating is the process of gradually exposing individuals to the feelings associated with the traumatic incident in a controlled and methodical manner. This allows the body to release energy and finish the physiological reactions that may have been interrupted during the first encounter.

Individuals can restore a feeling of agency over their narratives if they unravel the memories stored in their bodies. The body functions as a conduit via which the memories of the past are communicated and, in the end, altered. Individuals learn to explore their interior environment with curiosity, compassion, and resilience as a result of this process, which paves the way for healing to occur.

Exploring Sensations and Emotions

Somatic Landscape: The Language of Sensations

The investigation of sensations serves as the foundation of somatic therapy as a practice since they are the medium through which the body conveys its knowledge. The raw data of our physical experience and sensations comprise a spectrum of feelings ranging from faint vibrations to powerful and tangible experiences. Sensations can be triggered by a wide variety of stimuli in the body. Sensations are viewed as messengers in the context of somatic therapy, which aims to gain insights into the inner workings of the body-mind complex.

Tracking and Noticing

Tracking sensations involves cultivating a heightened awareness of the body's responses, whether in stillness or movement. It is an attunement to the ever-changing landscape of sensations, much like tuning in to the body's internal radio frequency. Practitioners of Somatic Therapy guide individuals to notice shifts in temperature, tension, pulsations, or other bodily sensations, providing valuable information about the individual's internal state.

The art of noticing is not merely observational; it is participatory. By actively engaging with sensations, individuals develop a more intimate relationship with their bodies. This process is integral to the therapeutic journey, fostering self-discovery and creating a bridge between conscious and unconscious aspects of the self.

Emotions as Embodied Expressions

Emotions are viewed as embodied manifestations rather than only cognitive experiences in the field of somatic therapy. Emotions are experienced feelings that appear in the body as well as the intellect. Think about the "pit in the stomach" that comes with anxiety or the "lightness in the chest" that comes with happiness. For those practicing somatic therapy, these physical manifestations of emotion are significant sources of knowledge.

Examining emotions within a somatic framework entails becoming aware of the physical experiences that correspond with various emotional states. It's a call to embrace the physical texture of feelings, enabling people to identify, label, and eventually control their emotional experiences through their bodies. People who go through this process will be more emotionally intelligent because they will have a more sophisticated knowledge of how emotions and bodily experiences interact.

Key Techniques in Somatic Therapy

- *Grounding and Centering Exercises*

Individuals are given the tools necessary to cultivate a feeling of stability and presence via the use of Somatic Therapy's basic practices, which include grounding and centering exercises. Connecting with the physical sensations of touch with the earth or another sturdy surface is an important part of the grounding process, which helps one become more rooted in the here and now. This technique might be very beneficial for people who are experiencing feelings of being overwhelmed or detached.

Bringing awareness to the center of the body, typically the region around the abdomen or the heart is the primary goal of the centering exercises. Individuals can build a sense of balance and inner stability when they attune themselves to this center axis. These exercises provide a foundation of safety and support, laying the footing for further somatic exploration and laying the groundwork for future somatic research.

- *Breathwork for Emotional Regulation*

The importance of the breath in Somatic Therapy cannot be overstated. It acts as an essential link between the aware and unconscious components of the body. Breathwork is not only about the act of breathing; rather, it is a dynamic process that involves attuning to the rhythm, depth, and quality of the breath as it mimics the emotional landscape. Breathwork is a component of somatic therapy.

Individuals have the opportunity to access a direct route to the regulation of their nervous system through the use of conscious breathing techniques such as diaphragmatic breathing or longer exhales. For instance, breathing in and out more slowly and deliberately can stimulate the parasympathetic nervous system, which in turn helps to promote relaxation and a sensation of peace. Breathwork is a strong technique for emotional regulation because it enables individuals to navigate and modify their emotional experiences by consciously engaging with their breath. This allows individuals to feel more in control of their emotions.

- ***Movement and Expression for Release***

The practice of somatic therapy acknowledges the innate value of the body's movement as an entry point to the processes of letting go and finding one's voice. Movement is not just a physical activity, but also a way of accessing and releasing energy as well as emotions that have been held. Movement may become a language through which the body communicates and processes events. This can happen in a variety of ways, including through mild stretches, spontaneous dancing, or expressive arts.

The process of releasing tension via movement does not have a specific objective in mind; rather, it is an investigation into the impulses and rhythms of the body. People are encouraged to move in ways that feel genuine and nourishing, which helps to promote a sense of release from the typical patterns of tension or limitation that they may have developed. Individuals can embody their stories by moving their bodies and expressing themselves, changing the somatic residue left over from previous events into a source of power and energy.

• *Integration of Mindfulness Practices*

The practice of mindfulness, which has its origins in contemplative traditions, is intertwined with all aspects of somatic therapy. The practice of mindfulness entails training oneself to become aware of their feelings, emotions, and ideas in the current moment without passing judgment on them. Mindfulness is used in somatic therapy as a bridge between the conscious and unconscious realms, giving people the ability to view their internal environment with both curiosity and compassion.

Body scans, in which individuals methodically bring attention to different regions of the

41

body, are one example of a mindfulness practice that may be included in somatic therapy. Another example is mindful movement, in which attention is integrated into the flow of various physical activities. These techniques strengthen the link between one's bodily awareness and mindfulness, which in turn fosters a relationship that is more integrated and harmonious with one's own subjective experience.

- *Embodied Practices in Psychotherapy*

Somatic Therapy is a comprehensive approach that may be used in a wide variety of therapeutic methods. This means that it is not limited to any one particular technique. Recognizing the body as an active participant in the therapeutic process is required for the successful integration of somatic activities into psychotherapy. A journey of self-discovery and healing may be created by a joint effort between the client and the therapist as the client is guided through the exploration of sensations, emotions, and movement patterns.

It is important to recognize that psychological and physiological processes are intertwined, and the integration of somatic approaches into psychotherapy does just that. Individuals can access deeper levels of experience, strengthening the therapeutic journey and encouraging transformation that is more permanent when they engage both their bodies and their minds.

- ***Empowering Self-Care Practices***

Somatic therapy gives people the tools they need to take their somatic practices outside of the therapy space and into their everyday lives, where they may serve as a kind of self-care. Moments of mindfulness, breathwork with intention, and brief grounding exercises may become tools for managing the obstacles of daily life. When people work on developing their somatic awareness, they build up a pool of resources that can be tapped into to foster resilience, well-being, and a sense of embodied vitality in themselves.

GROUNDING AND CENTERING EXERCISES

Exercises that focus on grounding and centering the body serve as core practices in the field of somatic therapy. These exercises provide participants with a direct link to the here and now as well as a stable platform on which to build future investigations. This in-depth investigation will delve into the complexities of grounding and centering, as well as their integration with breathwork for emotional regulation, the emancipatory power of movement and expression, and their role in comprehending trauma and stress within the context of the somatic experience.

Grounding and Centering: Foundations of Presence

- ### *The Essence of Grounding*

Individuals are encouraged to build a conscious connection with the Earth to root themselves in the here and now via the practice of grounding, which is a form of meditation. The practice of grounding in Somatic Therapy is more than just a physical activity; rather, it is a process that engages the full body-mind complex. It is a method for bringing surplus energy down to earth, establishing stability, and producing a feeling of security.

Many grounding exercises begin by directing the participant's attention to the sensation of making touch with the earth. This might be sensing the support provided by the feet on the floor, the weight of the body while seated in a chair, or the texture of the ground below. Individuals can develop a sense of rootedness and presence by cultivating this deliberate connection with their surroundings, which leads to the initiation of a conversation between the two.

- ### *The Role of Centering*

Drawing attention to the center of the body—typically the region surrounding the stomach or the heart—is the goal of centering, which is closely related to anchoring. The center is seen as a location of equilibrium, both energetically and physically. By helping people tune into this middle axis, centering exercises foster an inner feeling of alignment and stability.

Finding one's center is especially helpful when people are feeling disoriented, overburdened, or cut off. Focusing on the center allows people to realign their internal compass and tap into a stable source that provides a basis for additional somatic inquiry.

Breathwork for Emotional Regulation

- ## *Conscious Breathing and Emotional Regulation*

In Somatic Therapy, breathwork is a dynamic activity that extends beyond simple breathing reflexes. It entails using the breath as a means of conscious interaction between the body's aware and unconscious parts. Through deliberate breathing exercises, breathwork is a potent technique for emotional regulation that enables people to navigate and modify their emotional experiences.

Extended exhalations and diaphragmatic breathing are examples of conscious breathing techniques that have a direct impact on the autonomic nervous system. Through activating the parasympathetic nervous system, these exercises facilitate tranquility and relaxation. The breath becomes a dependable anchor in the context of emotional regulation, giving people a tool to manage the ups and downs of their internal emotional landscape.

- **Embodied Breath: A Mirror of Emotional States**

In somatic therapy, the breath is viewed as an embodiment of emotional experiences that may be expressed via the body. Various states of mind are each related to a certain rhythm of breathing. As an illustration, the symptoms of anxiety may include shallow and quick breathing, whereas the symptoms of grief may include slow and deep breathing. Individuals can acquire insight into their emotional experiences and cultivate a more embodied and nuanced grasp of their internal environment by tuning into the intricacies of the breath and attending to them.

Breathwork is not only useful for the management of emotions, but it is also an effective method for developing a more profound connection with one's physical self. People can establish a conversation with their somatic selves and build a bridge between their conscious and unconscious portions by bringing awareness to their breathing. This comprehensive approach to breathwork strengthens the therapeutic journey, allowing clients a road to greater self-awareness and emotional resilience in the process.

Movement and Expression for Release

- ### *The Power of Movement as a Somatic Language*

Movement is seen as a language by somatic therapists because it is the primary means by which the body communicates and makes sense of its experiences. Movement is not only an activity that takes place on the body; rather, it is a dynamic manifestation of the inner landscape. Movement may become a powerful instrument for releasing pent-up emotions and discovering more about oneself, whether it's done consciously through exercises or spontaneously through dance or expressive arts.

Movement activities in somatic therapy are not prescriptive but rather encourage individuals to investigate their one-of-a-kind bodily manifestations. Utilizing the body's inherent drive for motion as a method for releasing pent-up energy, alleviating muscle tension, and fostering a feeling of vigor is the goal of many forms of exercise. Movement is a liberating power that goes beyond verbal language and provides a direct conduit to the physical discharge of repressed emotions and experiences. Movement is a force that surpasses verbal communication.

- ***Expressive Modalities: Giving Voice to Emotions***

In addition to the physical act of moving one's body, individuals can verbalize their feelings via the use of expressive modalities such as music, painting, and dance. These modalities are not about creative competence in the physical environment; rather, they are about the process of expression itself. An individual will participate in a non-verbal conversation with their internal world whenever they create art, whether it be in the form of scribbling on paper, dancing to music, or producing art on the spur of the moment.

Expressive modalities act as vehicles for the discharge of feelings that may be difficult to describe verbally and serve as outlets for those feelings. Individuals are allowed to externalize and see their inner environment using the creative process, which acts as a mirror for the bodily experience. This technique is intrinsically empowering, since it encourages a sense of agency and self-discovery on the part of the participant.

Understanding Trauma and Stress

- ### *Somatic View of Trauma*

A somatic perspective on trauma is used in somatic therapy, which recognizes that traumatic events are not only imprinted in the mind but also held in the body. Somatic therapy relies on this premise. In the context of the body, trauma is understood to be imperfect bodily reactions to events that are both overwhelming and potentially life-threatening. These unfinished reactions get stuck in the neurological system, which then leads to patterns of tension, hypervigilance, and dysregulation.

Exercises that focus on grounding and centering the body are an important component of trauma-informed somatic treatments. Individuals who may be navigating the aftereffects of trauma might benefit from a strong foundation that can be established by establishing a sense of safety through grounding. When individuals are confronted with the dissolving consequences of trauma, centering may become a useful tool for them to restore a feeling of agency and coherence in their lives.

- **Somatic Techniques for Trauma Resolution**

Somatic Experiencing is a form of trauma resolution that falls under the umbrella of Somatic Therapy. This model emphasizes the renegotiation of traumatic experiences by tapping into the body's natural knowledge. Titration, which refers to the process of gradually exposing individuals to the sensations associated with trauma, and pendulation, which refers to the process of moving between the activation of traumatic memories and the experience of safety and resourcefulness, are two of the fundamental principles of Somatic Experiencing.

Breathwork is an essential element of the Somatic Experiencing method, and its purpose is to calm the nervous system and release the pent-up energy that is associated with traumatic memories. Movement and expression can become channels via which individuals can release rigid patterns of tension and integrate the bodily remnants of traumatic experiences. The purpose of grounding and centering exercises in the context of trauma recovery is to act as tools that may be used to build a container of safety, stability, and agency.

- **Somatic Approaches to Stress Management**

Even while traumatic stress is the most extreme kind of stress, the effects of everyday stresses are still left behind in the body. When seen from a somatic perspective, stress is recognized to be a physiological reaction that has the potential to become habitual, which can then lead to chronic patterns of tension and dysregulation. Individuals now have a straightforward and easily accessible tool at their disposal for controlling their stress in the here and now: grounding and centering exercises.

Individuals are given the ability to regulate their nervous system during times of increased stress via the practice of breathwork, which transforms into a portable tool for stress management. Both physical movement and verbal expression can act as channels for the outflow of surplus energy, therefore reducing the buildup of stress in the physical body. Individuals can build resilience and boost their capacity to traverse stresses with more ease when they include these somatic activities in their day-to-day lives.

SOMATIC PERSPECTIVE ON TRAUMA

Not only can trauma, whether it be acute or chronic, leave indelible marks on the psyche, but it also leaves those marks on the very fabric of the body. The somatic perspective on trauma provides a more complex understanding of how the body stores, expresses and seeks closure for traumatic events. This inquiry will dive into the identification and management of stress reactions, trauma-informed somatic methods, and the development of embodied resilience in the face of traumatic experiences.

Recognizing and Addressing Stress Responses

- ### *The Somatic Nature of Stress*

The human experience is inherently characterized by stress, which may be defined as a physiological reaction that serves to mobilize resources to deal with adversity. Nevertheless, when stress is persistent or excessive, the normal processes that the body has for adapting to it can become dysregulated, resulting in a wide variety of physical and psychological symptoms. According to the somatic point of view, stress is not just a cerebral experience but is also profoundly ingrained in the reactions of the body.

To recognize stress reactions, one must first become attuned to the body's subtle and not-so-subtle signals, which it sends out in reaction to various stressors. The manifestation of these messages may take the form of tense muscles, altered breathing patterns, an elevated heart rate, or changes in digestive function. The somatic lens recognizes that responses to stress are not confined to the mind but are instead intertwined throughout the physiology of the body as a whole.

• *The Impact of Chronic Stress*

Persistent patterns of tension and dysregulation can develop as a result of chronic stress, whether this stress is caused by present living issues or by traumatic experiences from the past. The body can develop a tolerance for being in a state of heightened awareness, which can lead to an endless feedback cycle of stress reactions. This prolonged activation of the stress response system can contribute to physical problems such as headaches, digestive troubles, and musculoskeletal discomfort. Additionally, it can contribute to emotional challenges such as anxiety and mood disorders.

When addressing stress reactions from a somatic point of view, it is important not just to recognize the symptoms, but also to investigate the underlying patterns that are occurring inside the body. This realization serves as the foundation for therapies that extend beyond the sphere of intellect, including the wisdom of the body in the process of regulating and healing.

Trauma-Informed Somatic Approaches

- ***Understanding Trauma Beyond the Mind***

The conventional approach to trauma, which is described as an event that is both overwhelming and potentially life-threatening, focuses largely on the use of psychological and cognitive frameworks. The somatic viewpoint, on the other hand, broadens our knowledge of trauma to include the physiological and sensory impressions that are left inside the body. Not only are traumatic events recalled in the mind, but they are also preserved in the neurological system, the muscles, and other somatic aspects.

69

The somatic techniques that are informed by trauma acknowledge the fact that traumatic experiences interrupt the natural flow of the body's reactions to stress. In the aftermath of traumatic experiences, the nervous system, which was developed to aid in the process of self-regulation, may become dysregulated. This dysregulation might show up as hypervigilance, dissociation, or an amplified startle response. These symptoms are the body's effort to cope with the unprocessed residues of traumatic events and can be a reflection of the body's attempts to cope.

Principles of Trauma-Informed Somatic Approaches

The following are some of the guiding concepts that are used in trauma-informed somatic therapies, which are used in the therapy process:

Safety and Stabilization: When dealing with trauma, it is of the utmost importance to create a feeling of safety. Exercises that focus on grounding and centering the body are frequently used to begin a sense of safety since these practices provide a solid foundation. These exercises equip individuals with the abilities necessary to negotiate situations of elevated stress or dissociation.

Titration and Pendulation: Titration is a method of administering therapy that entails dividing the healing process into smaller, more manageable parts. This method was developed in recognition of the fact that the overpowering nature of trauma calls for a cautious and step-by-step strategy. The process of pendulation entails going back and forth between the activation of painful memories and the sensation of being safe and capable. These concepts recognize the need to set boundaries and construct a safe environment to facilitate the processing of traumatic experiences.

Somatic Awareness: Gaining an awareness of one's own body's reactions and sensations is a necessary part of somatic awareness cultivation. Therapists assist clients in observing the minute changes in the body, which enables a more sophisticated comprehension of the somatic landscape. The layers of trauma held inside the body can be released by this knowledge.

Embodied Expression: Given the possibility that trauma will lead the mind-body link to break, embodied expression becomes crucial to healing. Through expressive modalities, breathwork, and movement, people can release the physical residue of trauma, allowing for a full sense of self.

- **_Breathwork in Trauma Resolution_**

Breathwork is essential in the context of trauma-informed somatic treatments. The breath is a physical means of balancing the neurological system and releasing pent-up energy from traumatic events. It acts as a link between the conscious and unconscious parts of the body.

Breathwork is used in trauma resolution models like Somatic Experiencing to assist people in renegotiating their connection with painful memories. By facilitating the completion of disrupted biological processes, conscious breathing aids the controlled release of trauma-related energy.

When used as a titration technique, breathwork allows people to push the boundaries of their comfort zones while still feeling comfortable. People who are attuned to their breath may find regions of limitation or tightness, which is a reflection of the bodily effects of trauma. The body's natural ability to self-regulate is activated via breathwork, providing a road to healing and reintegration.

- ***Movement as a Catalyst for Release***

A key element of trauma-informed somatic methods is movement, which acts as a catalyst for the release of energy and stress patterns that have been stuck. Trauma frequently results in immobility as the body prepares for traumatic events. Movement exercises, regardless of their intensity, help the body to reclaim its ability to move freely and expressively.

Movement in trauma recovery is not imposed; rather, it develops naturally from the person's lived experience. Therapists assist clients in investigating impromptu motions, gestures, or positions that emerge while they work with the physical aftereffects of trauma. Through this process, blocked energy may be released, habitual patterns can be broken, and a more harmonious relationship with the body can be developed.

- ## *Expressive Modalities for Externalizing Trauma*

Art, music, and dance are examples of expressive modalities that may be very effective in externalizing and processing traumatic events. Through the use of these modalities, people may communicate their inner selves nonverbally, overcoming the barriers posed by language and directly addressing the physical components of trauma.

Through creative processes, people can examine and explain their experiences in trauma-informed expressive arts treatments. People can externalize the inside landscape of trauma via dancing, painting, or sculpture, which promotes a sense of action and empowerment.

Traumatic memories can exist in the sensory and affective domains of the body and might be pre-verbal or non-verbal, according to the somatic viewpoint on trauma. To translate these somatic sensations into concrete forms of expression, expressive modalities serve as a bridge, fostering a more comprehensive and embodied trauma story.

Embodied Resilience: Cultivating Strength from Within

- ***Resilience as an Embodied Quality***

Embodied resilience is a trait that results from the union of the body and the mind, not only a cognitive ability. Developing resilience in the face of trauma entails negotiating the somatic landscape, regaining agency, and developing a cohesive connection with the body's reactions.

The foundation of embodied resilience is the understanding that the body has innate intelligence and the ability to self-regulate, even in the face of adversity. Exercises for centering and grounding people become instruments for building a stable basis from which they may explore and traverse their inner environment.

- **Integration of Trauma into the Narrative of Self**

Integrating one's experience of trauma into the overall story of who they are is a necessary component of embodying resilience. Individuals are taught to investigate how the body has adapted to and dealt with adversity rather than considering trauma as a static and solitary experience. This allows for a more holistic perspective on the effects of trauma. This approach entails understanding the impact that the trauma has on one's body while also appreciating the body's ability for change and growth.

Somatic techniques that are informed by trauma embrace a narrative of resilience that does not see the somatic experience as something apart from itself. Movement, breathwork, and expressive modalities all help to re-authoring the narrative, which enables individuals to externalize the bodily imprints of trauma and convert them into sources of strength and insight.

- ***Cultivating Mindfulness and Body Awareness***

Mindfulness, which has its origins firmly planted in somatic practices, emerges as an essential component of embodied resilience. Developing a non-judgmental awareness of the present moment, including one's physiological sensations, emotions, and thoughts, is an important step in the cultivation of mindfulness. Mindfulness can be utilized in the context of traumatic experiences as a method for attuning to the somatic landscape in a way that does not re-trigger overwhelming memories.

Individuals are encouraged to get intimately familiar with how their bodies react when they practice body awareness, a fundamental component of mindfulness in the somatic approach. This heightened awareness serves as a basis for detecting stress reactions, investigating the bodily intricacies of trauma, and establishing a relationship with oneself that is more embodied and robust.

- **Post-Traumatic Growth and Transformation**

Embodied resilience includes the possibility of post-traumatic growth and change in addition to the ability to adapt to trauma. The understanding that people may, by their somatic journey, emerge from horrific situations with renewed strengths, perspectives, and capabilities is known as post-traumatic development.

The somatic view on trauma recognizes that the body's reactions to trauma can include adaptive and transformational processes in addition to outward displays of anguish. Breathwork, expressive modalities, and movement all support the alchemical process of post-traumatic development by helping people integrate the knowledge and understanding they have obtained from their somatic inquiry.

BUILDING RESILIENCE THROUGH SOMATIC PRACTICES

The capacity to manage obstacles and recover quickly from setbacks is a trait known as resilience. This is a feature that may be developed via the use of practices that are both purposeful and embodied. The engagement of the body-mind complex in the process of self-discovery and change is one of the distinctive advantages offered by somatic therapies as a means of constructing resilience. This investigation will dig into the domains of establishing a positive body image, integrating somatic practices into everyday life, and encouraging mind-body connection as crucial factors in the road toward building resilience.

Cultivating a Positive Body Image

- ***Embarking on the Journey of Self-Appreciation***

Building resilience via somatic practices begins with fostering a healthy body image. The way we view and interact with our bodies has a big impact on our mental health, sense of self, and general ability to bounce back from setbacks in life. Through the comprehensive perspective offered by somatic techniques, people can set out on a path toward self-acceptance and respect.

- ***Unpacking Cultural Narratives***

The story that society has about body appearance frequently reinforces irrational

87

expectations and norms. Through questioning and dissecting these cultural myths, somatic practices help people realize that the body is a dynamic and expressive conduit of lived experience rather than just an object to be evaluated. Somatic inquiry allows people to take back control of their own story and move from criticism from others to self-compassionate discourse inside.

- **Embodied Practices for Body Awareness**

Somatic techniques cultivate a closer relationship with the body's sensations, motions, and expressions by increasing body awareness. By paying mindful attention to one's body, people may tune into their bodies' innate knowledge and avoid making assumptions about them from the outside world. By creating a sense of stability and presence, grounding and centering exercises—which are frequently used in somatic practices—become portals to a positive body image.

- **Movement as Celebration**

As a vital component of somatic inquiry, movement turns into a celebration of the capacities and individuality of the body. Somatic practices support people in moving in ways that are pleasurable and authentic rather than seeing movement as a way to meet social norms. Expressive movement, such as dance, yoga, or other forms, opens up channels for self-expression and cultivates a healthy relationship with the body as a source of joy and energy.

Integrating Somatic Techniques into Daily Life

- ## *Somatic Practices as Daily Rituals*

The advantages of strengthening resilience may be extended beyond formal practices and the venues in which they are delivered through the incorporation of somatic methods into everyday living. Exercises that help one become more grounded and centered, as well as breathwork and mindful movement, may all become rituals that are integrated into everyday routines. Amid all the pressures and expectations that life places on us, these rituals and routines may operate as a source of stability and relaxation.

- ### *Breathwork for Stress Management*

The core somatic practice of conscious breathwork provides an easily transportable instrument for the management of stress in day-to-day living. It is possible to combine straightforward practices, such as breathing with the diaphragm or pausing on purpose to become more mindfully aware of one's breath, into a wide variety of settings. Individuals may control their nervous systems and foster a sense of calm and resilience by paying attention to their breathing in response to stressful situations.

- ***Micro-Movements for Body Awareness***

It is not always necessary to do complex motions to cultivate somatic awareness; sometimes even the smallest movements may have a significant impact. Creating chances throughout the day to check in with the feelings experienced by the body can be accomplished by incorporating small minutes of body scanning or mild stretching. These little motions act as gentle prompts to be present in the body, which in turn helps to cultivate an ongoing connection with the physical experience.

- ### *Grounding Techniques for Presence*

In the middle of all the activities of everyday life, grounding methods, which have their origins in somatic practices, serve as a concrete anchor. Whether it's feeling the support of the feet on the ground while attending a meeting or taking a minute to connect with the breath before tackling a difficult activity, grounding is a skill that may be used to retain presence and stability in the face of the fluctuations that come with life.

Mind-Body Integration

• *The Unity of Body and Mind*

The integration of the mind and body is one of the primary focuses of somatic practices, which emphasize the interdependence of mental and physical health. The potential for resilience is not limited to only one's cognitive abilities; rather, it is profoundly ingrained in the very fabric of the body. Integrating the mind and body means acknowledging that one's ideas, feelings, and sensations experienced in the body are all closely connected and that developing resilience entails achieving a balance between these three aspects of one's experience.

- ***Somatic Awareness as a Gateway***

Developing somatic awareness is the first step toward mind-body integration. People can learn to watch ideas and feelings as they show up in their bodies through exercises like body scans. By bridging the gap between the somatic and cognitive domains, this awareness promotes a more comprehensive sense of self.

- ***Mindfulness as a Daily Practice***

For mind-body integration, mindfulness a key element of somatic approaches—becomes a daily habit. People develop a non-judgmental awareness of the present moment through formal meditation or casual periods of focused attention. Being mindful enables one to observe thoughts and feelings without becoming sucked into them, which promotes resilience and calmness.

- **Somatic Psychotherapy for Holistic Healing**

Recognizing the importance of the body in the healing process, somatic psychotherapy combines somatic methods with conventional therapeutic approaches. By assisting clients in examining the relationships between ideas, feelings, and physical experiences, therapists build a comprehensive framework for recovery. When people realize how intertwined their experiences are, resilience grows as a result of this mind-body integration in the therapeutic setting.

- ***Embodied Decision-Making***

By analyzing options using somatic signals, mind-body integration improves decision-making processes. Instead of depending exclusively on logical reasoning, people tune into their body's felt sense. Using the body's wisdom as a guide, this embodied decision-making method promotes a more genuine and in-tune way of handling life's challenges.

BRIDGING COGNITIVE AND SOMATIC APPROACHES

The convergence of somatic and cognitive techniques signifies a comprehensive worldview that acknowledges the complex interplay between the body and mind. This thorough examination will focus on promoting holistic well-being within the framework of somatic therapy, enhancing emotional intelligence through somatic awareness, and analyzing the various applications of somatic techniques in diverse contexts. It will also explore the synergies between these approaches.

Enhancing Emotional Intelligence through Somatic Awareness

- ### *The Symbiosis of Emotions and the Body*

The somatic landscape is intrinsically tied to emotional intelligence, which is the capacity to identify, comprehend, and regulate one's own emotions in addition to empathizing with others. Emotions are dynamic processes that materialize in the body as feelings, movements, and physiological reactions; they are not static events that occur only in the mind. Enhancing emotional intelligence, somatic awareness serves as a doorway to understanding the embodied basis of emotions.

- ***Somatic Practices for Emotional Regulation***

By being attuned to the body sensations that are connected with particular emotions, one may build a bridge between the cognitive and the somatic domains through the practice of somatic awareness. Individuals are given the tools necessary to successfully regulate their emotions when they participate in grounding and centering exercises, which are essential components of somatic practices. People can manage the complexities of their emotional experiences and cultivate a more nuanced and embodied awareness of themselves when they establish a connection with the present moment through their bodies.

• *Embodied Emotional Resilience*

The development of embodied emotional resilience can be enhanced by the use of somatic activities. People learn to approach their feelings with inquiry and an attitude of acceptance rather than considering them as something disruptive or overwhelming. During the process of emotionally exploring oneself, one's body takes on the role of a guide, providing information on the subtle shifts and patterns that are linked with the various emotional states. Because it is based on bodily awareness, this embodied resilience helps individuals to traverse the intricacies of their emotional experiences with more comfort and adaptability.

Holistic Well-being and Somatic Therapy

- ***Somatic Therapy as a Holistic Approach***

The integration of a person's physical, emotional, mental, and spiritual states into their overall state of health is what holistic well-being refers to. The emerging field of somatic therapy is an integrative mode of treatment that acknowledges the inextricable link between the human body and the mind. Somatic therapy, in contrast to treatments that concentrate only on cognitive processes, recognizes that the body is an active partner in the processes of healing and self-discovery, and treats it as such.

• *Attuning to the Body's Wisdom*

The practice of somatic therapy entails developing an awareness and receptivity to the body's wisdom as a storehouse of knowledge and insight. Individuals are led through an exploration of the somatic landscape by therapists, which helps them peel back the layers of tension, sensations, and emotions that are held inside the body. Exercises that focus on grounding and centering the body and mind serve as basic tools for building a sense of safety and presence, providing a framework for the investigation of holistic well-being.

- **Integration of Somatic and Verbal Processing**

In therapy, the integration of verbal and bodily processing enhances the breadth and depth of the therapeutic process. Somatic exploration offers a non-verbal means of expressing and processing events, whereas verbal processing enables people to convey their ideas and feelings. Combining the two approaches results in a more thorough and all-encompassing therapy procedure that addresses the various facets of well-being.

- **Trauma-Informed Holistic Healing**

The foundation for recovery that is provided by somatic therapy, in particular techniques that are trauma-informed, is comprehensive.

105

Not only are traumatic events etched into one's psyche, but they are also stored inside one's physical body. The somatic imprint of traumatic experiences is acknowledged in somatic therapy, and the tools it gives for renegotiating the impact of overwhelming events are provided. During the healing process, grounding, centering, and breathwork can become crucial components of trauma-informed somatic methods. This can help promote a sense of safety as well as a sense of empowerment.

Applications of Somatic Therapy

- ### *Individual Psychotherapy*

Somatic techniques provide a specific and nuanced investigation of the client's interior landscape in individual psychotherapy. Exercises for centering and grounding lay the groundwork for the therapeutic process, while somatic approaches like movement and breathwork offer pathways for self-awareness and recovery. By engaging the mind and body in the process of change, the integration of somatic and cognitive processes improves the efficacy of individual treatment.

• *Group Therapy and Expressive Arts*

There are many uses for somatic therapy in group settings, especially in expressive arts settings. Expressive modalities such as dance and movement may be effective instruments for promoting interpersonal relationships, communication, and group healing. Members of the group participate in somatic activities that promote self-expression, empathy, and the investigation of common somatic sensations. This cooperative strategy aids in the development of a caring community that is not limited by language.

- **Stress Management and Corporate Wellness**

For those juggling the rigors of the workplace, somatic approaches offer useful tools in the context of stress management and corporate wellness initiatives. In the workplace, techniques such as breathwork, mindfulness, and movement become accessible tools for managing stress reactions and fostering well-being. In corporate environments, somatic therapy recognizes the connection between physical and mental health, promoting an environment that prioritizes workers' overall well-being.

• *Sports Psychology and Performance Enhancement*

Sports psychology has benefited from the use of somatic treatment, which has improved athletes' performance. Somatic activities are employed by athletes to enhance their body-mind synchronization, attention, and resilience. Exercises that focus on centering and grounding yourself can be quite helpful in keeping your calm under pressure. Sports psychology has included somatic approaches to acknowledge the embodied character of athletic performance and the relationship between the body and mind.

SOMATIC THERAPY IN PSYCHOTHERAPY

Within the field of psychotherapy, the practice of somatic therapy offers a novel viewpoint that acknowledges the close relationship that exists between the human body and the mind. Within the context of psychotherapy, this in-depth investigation will delve into the application of somatic approaches in stress management, the integration of somatic practices for self-care, and the nuanced consideration of challenges and ethical considerations within the context of somatic therapy.

Somatic Approaches in Stress Management

- ### *The Physical Reaction to Stress*

Stress is a ubiquitous feature of the human condition, and its implications extend beyond the cognitive domain. The body reacts to stress by undergoing physiological changes, tensing muscles, and changing breathing patterns since it is a storehouse of life events. Somatic therapy is an integrated approach to stress management by recognizing the embodied character of stress and providing techniques to control both psychological and physiological reactions.

- *Using Breathwork as a Physical Aid*

Breathwork is a vital somatic skill for stress management. The body's conscious and unconscious parts can be connected through deliberate and aware interaction with the breath. To control the autonomic nervous system, somatic therapists assist patients in experimenting with different breathwork methods including diaphragmatic breathing or prolonged exhalations. People can use breathwork as an easily transportable and available technique to modify their stress reactions in real-time.

- ## *Stability via Centering and Grounding*

Exercises that center and ground the body are fundamental somatic activities that are essential for managing stress. Developing a conscious connection with the earth entails grounding, which is frequently accomplished by sensing one's feet's support. By focusing on the body's middle axis, centering promotes inner stability. When combined, these techniques give people a solid base on which to ground themselves in the here and now, providing a feeling of security and fortitude in the face of adversity.

- *Somatic Methods for Releasing Stress*

A variety of treatments are introduced in somatic therapy to relieve the body's stored tension and stress. Exercises that involve movement, like somatic experience or mindful stretching, offer ways to let go of extra energy. The innate propensity of the body to move is utilized to encourage calm and reestablish equilibrium. People who use somatic techniques go beyond cognitive ways to experience a journey of self-regulation and stress release.

Somatic Practices for Self-Care

- ### *Self-Care Rituals Embodied*

The relevance of integrating somatic activities into self-care routines is emphasized by somatic therapy. When incorporated into everyday routines, grounding, and centering exercises provide anchors that people may use for self-care moments. These exercises offer a concrete and approachable way to promote self-awareness, resilience, and general well-being.

- ***Using Body Scan Meditation to Reflect on Oneself***

A somatic technique called body scan meditation encourages people to methodically scan their bodies for stress points and feelings by paying focused attention to every aspect of their body. Through self-reflection and self-awareness, this practice helps people develop a stronger bond with their physical experiences. Body scan meditations serve as instruments for self-care, providing pockets of stillness and awareness amidst the stresses of everyday life.

- **Expressive Techniques for the Release of Emotions**

Incorporating expressive modalities like art, dance, or music into self-care routines is encouraged by somatic therapy. These modalities serve as channels for the release and expression of emotions, giving people imaginative ways to traverse their inner landscapes. By enabling people to externalize and process emotions in a non-verbal and bodily way, expressive somatic techniques help people feel more empowered.

- **Physical Self-Control for Emotional Sturdiness**

For emotional resilience, somatic self-regulation—which includes exercises like

118

movement and breathwork—becomes a crucial part of self-care. People acquire the ability to identify early indicators of stress or emotional dysregulation and use physical techniques to realign their nervous system. By taking a proactive stance towards self-regulation, people can improve their emotional resilience and become more adept at navigating the complicated emotional landscape.

Challenges and Ethical Considerations

- ## *Handling Opposition and Unease*

Although somatic therapy has the potential to be transformational, it can also cause resistance or discomfort, especially in those who are not used to talking about the bodily aspects of their experiences. To effectively manage resistance, therapists must provide a secure and encouraging therapeutic atmosphere. People are more comfortable with the somatic components of treatment when somatic activities are introduced gradually and their purpose and potential benefits are communicated clearly.

- ***Making Certain Informed Consent***

When using somatic techniques in psychotherapy, informed permission must be obtained comprehensively. People must comprehend the nature of somatic activities, as well as any potential advantages and any emotional or physical side effects. Therapists need to make sure that clients feel empowered to voice any concerns or desires about using somatic approaches, as well as to clearly explain the intended somatic treatments.

- ***Honoring Limitations and Sensitivity to Trauma***

In somatic therapy, it is crucial to honor each person's limits and psychological sensitivity. Personal space and comfort are important concerns while engaging in certain somatic activities that require physical contact or proximity. To ensure that somatic therapies are customized to promote safety and prevent re-traumatization, therapists need to be aware of the distinct needs and histories of each client. Titration and pendulation are given priority in trauma-informed somatic techniques, such as those found in Somatic Experiencing, to enable people to engage in somatic exploration at a manageable speed.

- **Combining Verbal and Somatic Processing Ethically**

Therapists must exercise caution while integrating verbal and physical processing because of power dynamics in the therapeutic alliance. Although somatic activities can further the exploration, therapists need to be mindful of the patient's comfort zone and preparedness. Transparent communication on the goal and methodology of somatic therapies promotes a therapeutic dynamic that is both cooperative and empowering.

POTENTIAL CHALLENGES IN SOMATIC WORK

Somatic work has transformational possibilities in therapeutic settings because it emphasizes the connection between the mind and body. Like any treatment strategy, it has some potential drawbacks, though. The intricacies of negotiating moral standards for somatic practitioners and emphasizing client empowerment via informed permission will be examined in this investigation.

Ethical Guidelines for Somatic Practitioners

- ## *Clients' safety and wellbeing*

In somatic treatment, safeguarding clients' safety and well-being is one of the main ethical issues. Physical contact, movement, and other therapies are examples of somatic techniques, and their practitioners must be sensitive to the distinct requirements and comfort zones of each client. Upholding ethical norms in somatic work requires setting clear limits, clarifying objectives, and following up with clients regularly to learn about their experiences.

- **Practices Informed by Trauma**

Since somatic work frequently explores the embodied parts of trauma, practitioners need to develop trauma-informed approaches. This entails being aware of how somatic therapies may affect people who have experienced trauma in the past and modifying methods to put safety first and reduce the chance of re-traumatization. Trauma-informed somatic treatment necessitates an understanding of titration and pendulation principles as well as respecting the individual's pace in somatic inquiry.

- **Observing Sensitivities to Culture**

Practitioners need to understand the cultural environment in which their clients live since somatic practice is not culturally neutral. Cultural differences can influence how people feel about touching, expressing themselves physically, and sharing personal space. Clinicians need to take a culturally sensitive approach to somatic therapies, honoring different viewpoints on the body and its function in therapy.

- **Maintaining Privacy in Somatic Investigation**

Confidentiality preservation is a fundamental ethical principle of all therapeutic methods, including somatic treatment. The somatic component often includes the exploration of very personal and physical experiences. Practitioners must use the utmost caution and confidentiality while managing any documents or information related to somatic therapies to preserve client privacy.

- **Ongoing Professional Improvement**

Somatic practitioners are morally obligated to pursue continuous professional development. Providing high-quality treatment requires staying current with new research, evolving techniques, and moral dilemmas in the ever-evolving field of somatics. Ongoing training helps practitioners improve their skills, deepen their understanding of morality, and apply the most recent research-based techniques to their somatic work.

Client Empowerment and Informed Consent

- ### *Teamwork in Making Decisions.*

Ethical somatic practice is centered on client empowerment. It is recommended that practitioners use a collaborative approach, involving clients in joint decision-making concerning the objectives, techniques, and sequencing of somatic treatments. By allowing clients to actively shape their treatment path, this collaborative style fosters a sense of agency and autonomy.

- ### *Open and honest dialogue on somatic methods.*

A fundamental component of moral behavior in somatic work is informed consent. Practitioners are required to give customers thorough information regarding the nature of somatic treatments, their possible advantages, and any dangers or discomforts that may be involved. Clear communication builds a trustworthy therapeutic alliance and empowers clients to make educated decisions regarding their involvement in somatic therapies.

- **Respecting the Limits of the Client.**

In somatic work, it is crucial to acknowledge and respect the boundaries set by the client. This entails recognizing and modifying the strategy in response to any discomfort or resistance that clients may feel during somatic therapies. It is the responsibility of practitioners to establish a setting where clients feel comfortable communicating their limits and know that their choices will be honored.

- **Teaching Patients about Somatic Mechanisms.**

Practitioners should inform clients about the potential somatic processes they may encounter in addition to getting their permission. Psychoeducation about the mind-body link, the possibility of releasing emotions or memories held in the body, and the function of somatic therapies in promoting general well-being are all included in this. By demystifying the bodily experience, education helps clients feel less anxious or unsure.

* *Flexible treatment plans.*

Treatment strategies must be flexible to empower clients. Because somatic work is extremely customized, practitioners should be willing to modify their therapies in response to client's changing needs and preferences. Flexibility helps clients reach their specific therapy objectives and guarantees that the therapeutic process stays sensitive to the dynamic character of somatic inquiry.

Navigating Challenges and Ensuring Ethical Somatic Practice

- *Peer consultation and supervision.*

Practitioners in somatic work should actively participate in peer consultation and supervision to manage the possible obstacles. Practitioners can reflect on their therapeutic practice, get advice on difficult patients, and get input on their somatic therapies during routine supervision meetings. Through the development of a cooperative community of practitioners who can exchange insights and work together to resolve ethical conundrums, peer consultation enhances the educational process even further.

- **Code of Ethics for Professionals.**

Somatic practitioners need to understand and abide by the professional code of ethics that applies to their particular discipline. In any somatic discipline—be it body-oriented psychotherapy, somatic psychology, or another—knowing the values and ethical standards established by pertinent professional associations is essential. When making moral judgments in their somatic work, practitioners might use these codes of ethics as guiding principles.

- **Frequent introspection.**

To sustain ethical somatic practice, regular self-reflection is essential. It is important for practitioners to consistently assess their prejudices, cultural presumptions, and any countertransference responses about somatic therapies. Practitioners become more conscious of their somatic sensations and how they could affect their interactions with clients through self-reflection.

- **Handling Countertransference in Somatic Practices.**

In practitioners, somatic activity can elicit severe bodily countertransference reactions. Practitioners must acknowledge and deal with their bodily reactions to the experiences of their clients. To explore and process countertransference reactions, supervision, and individual therapy can be helpful tools.

This helps to guarantee that practitioners keep a distinct and unambiguous viewpoint during somatic sessions.

CONCLUSION

To sum up, the investigation of somatic therapy in the context of psychotherapy uncovers a transforming methodology that addresses the complex interaction between the mind and body. Given the ethical constraints and the need for informed consent in empowering clients, a nuanced and considered approach must be used when utilizing somatic work due to its possible problems.

For somatic practitioners, ethical guidelines act as a compass, helping them to navigate the challenges of cultural sensitivity, safety, and trauma sensitivity. Upholding the ethical criteria that serve as the cornerstone of ethical somatic work requires a high priority on protecting clients' safety and well-being, implementing trauma-informed methods, honoring cultural sensitivities, and protecting client confidentiality. The ethical foundation of somatic therapy is also influenced by ongoing professional development and a dedication to remaining up-to-date on changing practices.

A major theme that comes through is client empowerment, emphasizing the value of open communication, group decision-making, and respecting client boundaries. Not only does informed consent become an essential procedure, but it also becomes a dynamic process where clients actively shape their treatment path. A therapeutic relationship built on mutual respect and trust can be achieved through educating clients about somatic processes, encouraging flexibility in treatment plans, and creating an atmosphere in which clients feel empowered to express their boundaries.

Practitioners must take a proactive and thoughtful approach due to the possible obstacles associated with somatic practice. Through continuous self-reflection, peer consultation, and supervision, practitioners may investigate their bodily reactions, resolve countertransference, and improve their abilities over time. To engage in ethical somatic practice, practitioners must be sensitive to both their own developing understanding of the mind-body connection and the needs of their clients.

In the end, moral somatic practice serves as the cornerstone around which the therapeutic journey of somatic therapy is built. It is this dedication to moral principles, client empowerment, and continuous introspection that enables somatic practitioners to meet obstacles with tact and expertise. Somatic therapy is revealed as a comprehensive and holistic technique that encourages people to explore the rich terrain of their embodied existence, promoting healing, resilience, and transformation in this blend of ethical considerations and client-centered approaches.